Memory DayByDay

*A New Model of Caring*

## The Dementia Friends Handbook

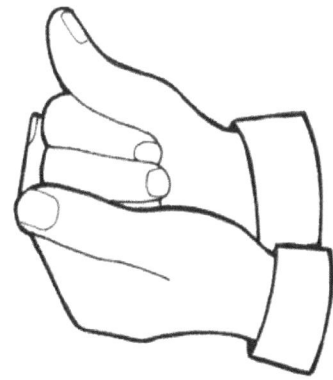

*I'm a Dementia Friend because I want to help.*

# The Dementia Friends Handbook

# The Dementia Friends Handbook

## By

## Patricia Bruketta, MSN, NP

First Edition
2015

I dedicate this book to Tommy Ryan who once told me
growing up in Little Rock, Arkansas
was the happiest time of his life.

Tom,
You were
a supportive friend to those who knew you
a generous, loving father for Tegan & Travis
a wonderful, gentle husband and my best friend

# Table of Contents

# Acknowledgement

I want to thank the board members of Memory DayByDay for their dedication to helping my work come to light: Scott Abramson, Nancy Hoffman, Michael McDonald, Patrick Sheridan.

The artwork on the cover was designed by my sister, Ann. The hands are signing "help" in American Sign Language. She is one of the most resourceful and creative artists I have ever known.

I was inspired by a talk I heard by Nicole Batsche who came all the way from King's College, London to speak at the dementia conference in San Diego, California in May 2014. She gave a powerful and timely talk called "The Stigma of Dementia". It was the first time I heard about inviting people to become Dementia Friends. Jaime Tyrone, owner of the non-profit company called B.A.B.E.S., encouraged me to move forward with my dream.

I want to thank Mr. Ward Pynn who encouraged me to register Memory DayByDay as a nonprofit corporation. He knows how much I want to reach out to everyone regardless of their financial situation.

I thank my many friends who acted as editors: Rebecca and Bruce Oatman, Anne Morrissette, Dolores Sirca, Betty and Pete Foott, Christin and Dave Anderson, and Pat Sheridan.

There are so many others I need to thank. I hope you know who you are. I also acknowledge and thank those who will read this book and become Dementia Friends. We need you and I'm grateful you have decided to act.

# Preface

I am writing this book to help people learn how to assist people with dementia. The aim of this handbook is to help you become comfortable in talking to people with this disease.

My hope is people who work in retail, banks, churches, medical and dental clinics, and other work environments will read this book so they can help people with dementia who may become confused, lost, or separated from a friend or family member. After reading my book you will be able to increase the quality of life for people living with dementia.

My passion is to specifically help people diagnosed with Alzheimer's dementia before the age of 65. People with early-onset Alzheimer's dementia can be more aware of the disease process as is seen in the beautiful video produced in England. It can be seen on my website. I am in the process of creating a Dementia Friend video which will be shown on my website once it is done.

We need to support research that can help those living with dementia today so they can enjoy a meaningful life as well as research to find the cause and cure of this disease. It's vital they know they haven't been forgotten or dismissed.

If you live in the United States, go to my website, www.memorydaybyday.org, to get information about how to obtain the Dementia Friend kit. This book will be included in the kit to share with others.

Thank you
Tricia Bruketta, MSN, NP
Memory DayByDay
April 15, 2015

# Key Points

# Friendship

With a diagnosis of dementia the support of friends, as well as the family members, is vital to the person's sense of well-being.

It is usually expected that the family will be supportive. But when friends also remain present during this time, it means so much to the one with dementia because they know there is no obligation.

# Respect

Although many people with dementia lose the ability to speak, they become masters of the emotional life.

They can sense when they are not welcome or accepted. Not feeling respected, as an adult, can provoke agitation and adverse behavior coming from the negative feelings.

# Communication

Keep explanations about a situation simple, this helps the person understand and accept what is happening.

If people with dementia become agitated or verbally loud, it is very important to remain calm and present a reassuring manner.

They will respond to a positive manner, regardless of what is said. And the opposite is true: reassuring words said with anger or sarcasm will not be accepted.

The person with dementia takes approximately 60 seconds to respond to a question. So, it is important to give him time to process the first question and answer, before asking another question.

When language becomes confusing, then it is important to remember they are experts at reading nonverbal communication.

We all read our environment according to what we understand. We also respond with behaviors to what we think is happening to us. So, it is the same to someone with dementia. If they appear angry, then they have perceived something in the environment as negative, even if their perception isn't accurate. We need to address the feelings, not the words.

Bottom line
Keep it simple and stay calm

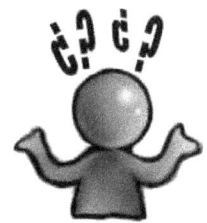

# Our own view of dementia

How we, the friends and family, view dementia is reflected in our interactions with our loved one.

Do we see only loss?

Do we believe that our relationship is supportive and makes a difference?

Are we willing to travel the road with the person, adapting our conversation and activity to stay in step with them?

Are we willing to step into their world that may seem to be strangely different?

# Introduction

This is a handbook to help people communicate comfortably with people diagnosed with dementia. There are many books that go into detail about the disease, diagnosis, and treatment. My book is going to stress practical ways to talk and work with people dealing with early-onset dementia. If you want detail information about the disease and treatment, there will be a resource list in Chapter Four and References.

Dementia is a general term for several conditions. The different types of dementia, as well as the different stages of Alzheimer's dementia, will be outlined in Chapter One so we can have a general idea of the disease and the process (symptoms) the person may be going through.

I found that people react to dementia like people react to cancer. I hear comments like:

"I don't know what to say to them."

"I don't visit because I think I make him nervous."

"I feel so sad because I remember what she used to be like."

We need to be aware of these feelings of inadequacy and sorrow in order to face this terrible disease honestly. We can each make a difference in the life of people with dementia by learning new skills and communication techniques to improve their quality of life. Our friends and family members will also need our support and friendship, especially as the disease progresses.

We can make a difference for the caregivers. Caregivers want their loved ones to be respected and treated with dignity, i.e. not to be dismissed or ignored. The caregiver wants to know that their loved one's behavior will be understood or, at least, tolerated, especially in public when the person with dementia may be more likely to be anxious and frightened.

In his book, *Dementia Reconsidered* (Kitwood, 1997), Tom Kitwood speaks about the personhood of the individual with dementia. He stresses the importance of continuing to respond to the person no matter how advanced the dementia. Many times people treat the person as an object, that is, something to be fed, clothed, and bathed. We need to learn how to speak and treat someone with dementia with respect, even in advanced stages. The Dementia Friends Handbook will provide some tools and ways to communicate so the personhood of each individual is preserved.

You may discover many different avenues of communication once you start. Maybe it will be customers who are confused about finding the restroom. If you know they have problem with verbal directions, then by walking them to the location of the restroom will help them feel understood and less anxious. For example, I went to a woodworking store and my husband needed to use the bathroom. The man behind the counter walked Tom to the bathroom and then came back and rang up my purchase. I felt he understood the situation and he helped me feel supported. Caregivers can feel helpless in public places when trying to run errands with their loved one. When there is the perception of no help or support, it can become overwhelming.

I would love to hear your stories of support and communication. You can send them to my email or write about it on my blog at www.memorydaybyday.org. With your feedback and contributions, we can advance the mission to make help caregivers and people with dementia remain part of the social fabric whether it is in stores, banks, churches, medical/dental offices and restaurants.

# Chapter One

Types of Dementia
Signs of Alzheimer's Dementia
Executive Functions

Dementia is an umbrella term under which there are different types and each has a unique presentation. Sometimes the person can have a mixed dementia that starts with one type and then acquires another.

Dementia is not just difficulty remembering things. Many times we all forget where we put our keys or to return a phone call. Memory loss in dementia is a matter of degree. Days may run together when we are on vacation, but a person with dementia believes it is winter in May because it is cold outside. They won't remember the actual year, even when reminded several times. They don't just forget where they put their keys, but put them in the refrigerator because "that's where they go."

In addition to memory loss, in dementia, there is also a problem with some aspect of an individual's executive functions. A definition given on the website www.minddisorders.com is the following:

> Executive functions are necessary for goal-directed behavior. They include the ability to initiate and stop actions, to monitor and change behavior as needed, and to plan future behavior when faced with novel tasks and situations. Executive functions allow us to anticipate outcomes and adapt to changing situations. The ability to form concepts and think abstractly is often considered components of executive function.

The website then further defines the executive functions by clearly delineating the tasks that are performed.

Executive function refers to a set of mental skills that are coordinated in the brain's frontal lobe. Executive functions work together to help a person achieve goals. Executive function includes the ability to:

  manage time and attention
  switch focus
  plan and organize
  remember details
  curb inappropriate speech or behavior
  integrate past experience with present action

With executive function affected, it becomes more apparent that the person is having difficulty with work, leisure activities, and social relationships. Initially, family and friends may think the behavior is caused by stress, depression, or anxiety. Eventually, the behavior and memory loss becomes so pronounced the family or close friends recommend the person see their medical provider. I recommend someone who knows the person with memory issues go with her to the doctor's office. Social behavior remains intact even with advanced dementia. The person will continue to answer social questions correctly. For example, the doctor may ask, "Are you sleeping well?" The patient will respond, "Yes, thank you for asking." When in reality, family members have found her wandering at night.

It's important to remember when the frontal lobe is affected the lack of initiative doesn't mean they are lazy or that they don't care.

They will say exactly what they are thinking, because the part of the brain that helps us with impulse control is no longer there. Once when Tom and I were in a restaurant, we passed a table with someone who was overweight. He asked me, "Why don't they exercise and lose weight?" I just replied, "I don't know. Maybe they don't have time." And then I changed the subject.

As mentioned at the beginning, dementia is an umbrella term for several different types of syndromes. The most common type is Alzheimer's dementia. The other types are Frontotemporal, Lewy body, Normal Pressure Hydrocephalus, Vascular, Huntington's, Parkinson, and AIDs. Frontotemporal dementia is characterized by behavioral changes. Lewy body, like Parkinson, has muscle and balance problems. Vascular dementia looks like the person is having mini-strokes followed with periods of stability until the symptoms worsen again.

Dementia is a frightening disease, especially if it happens to someone close to you. It is estimated there are two million people living with Alzheimer's dementia in the United States. Of those two million people, 5-10 % are living with early-onset Alzheimer's dementia. Most people think of dementia as a slowly progressive disease of the elderly. The reality is that 100,000-200,000 people are diagnosed before the age of 65.

Ten warning signs of dementia from Alzheimer's Association website: (Alzheimer's Association, 2014)

1. Memory loss that disrupts daily life

2. Challenges in planning or solving problems

3. Difficulty completing familiar tasks at home, at work, or at leisure.

4. Confusion with time and place

5. Trouble understanding visual images and spatial relationships

6. New problems with words in speaking or writing.

7. Misplacing things and losing ability to retrace steps

8. Decreased or poor judgment

9. Withdrawal from work or social activities

10. Changes in mood and personality

In the next chapter I will discuss some details about Alzheimer's Dementia. This is the most prevalent form of dementia and will most likely be encountered.

# Chapter Two

# Normal Aging vs Cognitive Impairment
# Stages of Alzheimer's disease

Many people may forget something from time to time because they are distracted or are trying to do several things at one time. I found a table developed by David Knopman, MD (American Medical Association, 1999, p. 4) that compares normal aging to someone with dementia.

| Typical Aging | Dementia |
| --- | --- |
| Independence in daily activities | Person becomes critically dependent on others for key independent living activities |
| Complains of memory loss but able to provide considerable detail regarding incidents of forgetfulness | May complain of memory problems only if specifically asked; unable to recall instances where memory loss was noticed |
| Patient is more concerned about alleged forgetfulness than are close family members | Close family members much more concerned about incidents of memory loss than patient |
| Recent memory for important events, affairs, conversations not impaired | Notable decline in memory for recent events and ability to converse |
| Occasional word finding difficulties | Frequent word finding pauses and substitutions |
| Does not get lost in familiar territory; may have to pause momentarily to remember way | Gets lost in familiar territory while walking or driving; may take hours to eventually return home |
| Able to operate common appliances even if unwilling to learn how to operate new devices | Becomes unable to operate common appliances; unable to learn to operate even simple new appliances |
| Maintains prior level of interpersonal skills | Exhibits loss of interest in social activities; exhibits socially inappropriate behaviors |
| Normal performance on mental status examinations, taking education & culture into account | Abnormal performance on mental status examination not accounted for by education or cultural factors. |

As we see, it is a matter of degree. Dementia is also disabling to the person involved. The normal routines are no longer "normal." Although, it has been shown that procedural memory remains intact for a longer period of time.

Procedural memory includes the memories we have been laying down all of our life. It is the act of brushing our teeth, riding a bicycle, or putting on our coat. Sometimes the person with dementia may not remember how to put the toothpaste on the toothbrush but once the act of brushing is started they proceed without assistance.

This is important to know in order to assist those with dementia remain independent in as many areas of their life as possible.

Several sources have developed charts in how to stage the disease progression. I found seven stages on the Alzheimer's Association website (Alzheimer's Association, 2014), five stages from several articles (Morris, 1993) (Hughes, Berg, Danziger, & al, 1982) (Heyman, Wilkinson, & Hurwitz, 1987) and finally three stages as presented by National Institute on Aging (Kathy Black, 2014, pp. 9-10). If you eliminate the stage in which there are no symptoms or mild memory loss without loss of daily functioning, then we come up with five stages. Mild cognitive impairment (MCI) is the stage before people start having problems with day to day life. Fifty percent of people diagnosed with MCI eventually develop Alzheimer's dementia. I have combined the various sources into one table listing N.I.A. first, then the neurologists, and finally Alzheimer's Association. They all bring out different aspects and help people understand the progression of the disease.

| References — Stages | NIA — Mild | Neurologists — Mild, 1+ | Alzheimer's — Mild cognitive decline |
|---|---|---|---|
| Memory | Memory loss | Moderate memory loss, more marked with recent events; defect interferes with everyday activities | Doctors may be able to detect memory or concentration problems; trouble remembering names when introduced to new people; forgetting material one has just read |
| Orientation | Confusion about the location of familiar places | Moderate difficulty with time relationships; oriented for space at examination, may have geographic disorientation elsewhere | |
| Executive functioning | Trouble handling money & paying bills; poor judgment leading to bad decisions | Moderate difficulty in handling problems, similarities, and differences; social judgement usually maintained | Trouble coming up with the right word or name; increased trouble with planning or organizing |
| Community affairs | Loss of spontaneity & sense of initiative | Unable to function independently at these activities but may be engaged in some; appears normal to casual inspection | Having noticeably greater difficulty performing tasks in social or work settings. |
| Home & hobbies | Longer to accomplish daily tasks | Mild but definite functional impairment at home; abandons more difficult chores, as well as hobbies and previous interests | Friends, family or co-worker begin to notice difficulties |
| Personal care, emotions | Mood & personality change; increased anxiety | Needs prompting | Losing or misplacing valuable objects |

| | | | |
|---|---|---|---|
| Personal care, emotions | Restlessness, agitation, anxiety, tearfulness, hallucination, delusion, paranoia, irritability | Require assistance in dressing, hygiene, maintaining personal effects | Becoming moody or withdrawn, especially in socially or mentally challenging situations |
| Home & hobbies | Problem recognizing friends & family members; repetitive statement or movements; occasional muscle twitches; perceptual-motor problems (trouble getting out of a chair or setting the table) | Only simple chores preserved; very restricted interests; poorly maintained | Greater difficulty performing complex tasks, such as planning dinner for guests, paying bills or managing finances |
| Community affairs | Difficulty coping with new or unexpected situations | No pretense at independent function outside the home; appears well enough to be accompanied to functions outside the home | |
| Executive functioning | Difficulty organizing thoughts & thinking logically; loss of impulse control | Severe impairment in handling problems, similarities, and differences; social judgment usually impaired | Impaired ability to perform challenging mental arithmetic |
| Orientation | Wandering, especially in late afternoon or at night | Severe difficulty with time relation-ships; usually disoriented to time, often to place | Forgetful-ness about one's own personal history |
| Memory | Increasing loss and confusion; shortened attention span; inability to learn new things | Severe memory loss; only well-learned material retained; new material rapidly lost | Forgetful-ness of recent events |
| **Stages** | **Moderate** | **Moderate, 2+** | **Moderate cognitive decline** |
| References | NIA | Neurologist | Alzheimer's |

| Stages | Alzheimer's — Moderately severe cognitive decline | Neurologists — Severe, 3+ | NIA — Severe |
|---|---|---|---|
| Memory | Gaps in memory & thinking are noticeable; can't remember schools they've attended; still remember significant details about themselves & their family | Severe memory loss; only fragments remain | |
| Orientation | Unable to recall their own address or telephone number; Become confuse about where they are or what day it is | Orientation to person only | |
| Executive functioning | Have trouble with less challenging mental arithmetic | Unable to make judgments or solve problems | |
| Community affairs | | No pretense at independent function outside the home; appears too ill to be taken to functions outside the home | |
| Home & hobbies | Begin to need help with day-to-day activities | No significant function in the home | Difficulty swallowing; increased sleeping; groaning, moaning or grunting |
| Personal care, emotions | Need help choosing proper clothing for the season or the occasion; require no assistance with eating or using the toilet | Require much help with personal care; frequent incontinence | Weight loss; seizures; skin infections; lack of bladder and bowed control |

| | Profound, 4+ | Terminal, 5+ | Severe cognitive decline | Very severe cognitive decline |
|---|---|---|---|---|
| Personal care, emotions | May attempt to dress or feed self, non-ambulatory without assistance; most incontinent | | Personality changes may take place and individuals need extensive help with daily activities; need help dressing properly; experience major changes in sleep patterns | Need help with eating & toileting; lose the ability to smile; swallowing impaired |
| Home & hobbies | Unable to participate meaning-fully in any hobby or home activity | Needs to be fed; is bedridden; incontinent | Have trouble remembering the name of a spouse or caregiver; Need help handling details of toileting, increase in incontinence | Lose ability to respond to their environment; to carry on a conversation & eventually control movement |
| Community affairs | Unable to participate meaning-fully in any social setting | | | |
| Executive functioning | Unable to follow even simple instructions or commands | Completely unable to engage in any activity | | |
| Orientation | Occasionally responds to own name | No recognition of self | Lose awareness of recent experiences as well as of their surroundings; tend to wander or becomes lost | May say words & phrases; lose ability to sit without support or hold their heads up; reflexes abnormal; muscles grow rigid |
| Memory | Even fragments of memory generally lost; memory testing made difficult by unintelligible or irrelevant speech | | Memory continues to worsen; remember their own name but have difficulty with their personal history | |
| **Stages** | **Profound, 4+** | **Terminal, 5+** | **Severe cognitive decline** | **Very severe cognitive decline** |
| References | Neurologist | | Alzheimer's | |

We can look at the last stages and feel fairly helpless. But there are new therapies now helping those in the late stages enjoy life. Music therapy is beginning to be used with positive effects as witnessed by the video of "Henry". I have a link to this video on my website (www.memorydaybyday.org) in the Memory Café section. I'm hoping to make use of this therapy in the Memory Cafés I open. It is a wonderful example of what Tom Kitwood (Kitwood, 1997) would refer to as "personhood". We learn about what this individual likes and then watch him wake up, as Dr. Sachs says on the video.

Even at the end of life there are moments the individual person, for a brief moment, connects with another human being. These moments are so fragile that we can miss them while we complete the tasks around us.

My husband was admitted to the hospital for an infection toward the end of his life. The nurses were kind but too busy to take the time needed to ask a question and wait for his answer. Every morning they would come in and say, "Good morning! Do you want to get out of bed? Are you ready for breakfast? Did you sleep well?" Three questions in a row with no time for him to say anything. It has been shown that it takes 60 seconds for someone with dementia to hear and respond to a question. Sometime, as an experiment, ask a question and then time 60 seconds on your watch and you will think that's a long time to wait.

One day after a procedure in which Tom had answered several questions I asked, the aide went and brought the nurse in to see that he could talk!

While the nurse was there, I asked a simple question, "Tom, how do you feel?" and I waited, keeping eye contact with him. He slowly said, "I'm scared." The nurse immediately tried to reassure him that they would take care of him. But in the following days, the rapid succession of questions did not stop, such as "How did you sleep? Are you ready to get up? Are you hungry?" And Tom again was silent, except when I would sit with him.

The reason to start the Dementia Friends movement and for the writing of this handbook is to help people learn how to treat people with dementia as people, i.e. human beings with feelings and physical sensations. Tom Kitwood noticed that many people treat people with dementia in an I-It relationship which occurs when the person with dementia is no longer seen as a person but a body to be washed, fed, clothed and put to bed. They stop interacting with them. I hope music therapy will catch on because it allows that silent person to come alive again to those around him. On the website, www.musicandmemory.org, they have training classes to promote the use in music therapy.

# Chapter Three

## Behavioral Expressions
## Communication Strategies

This chapter will cover many of the "problems" people with dementia eventually exhibit. How can the environmental and interpersonal factors become reflected in the behavior of someone with dementia?

If we weren't feeling so embarrassed at the time a loved one says or does something socially inappropriate, we would find the human mind is still trying to find ways to make sense of the world around it.

Instead of trying to help them "see reason", we could start by accepting them and trying to find the cause of the behavior. Telling someone with dementia what they said isn't right would be confusing to them, because they think it is right. The best book I read early on in my care of Tom was a book called, *Learning to Speak Alzheimer's* (Coste, 2003). I strongly urge anyone who wants to help people with dementia feel accepted to read Ms. Coste's book. She gives multiple examples of trying to see what the person with dementia is seeing. She then writes about changing the environment or phrasing a question to help the person feel comfortable again. This occurred multiple times with Tom but one short example will serve as an explanation.

Tom woke up one night at two o'clock in the morning. He woke me up when he sat up in bed and asked me, "Why is the train stopped?" I thought he had been dreaming so I first said, "It's okay, we're at home." Tom then asked, "OK, but shouldn't someone tell us why the train has stopped?" I asked, "So what type of engineer would take care of this problem?" He thought and replied, "a mechanical engineer." I then asked him about his father and grandfather who were both engineers, mechanical and civil respectively.

When I thought I had moved him past worrying about the train, he said, "This isn't right! Someone should let us know why the train is stopped!" Now he was getting angry. I said, as lightly as I could, "Well, we have a bed. So, why don't we go to sleep, let them fix the train and in the morning we will be where we are supposed to be!" He thought about it, "OK." He lay down and went back to sleep. I looked around our room and noticed the bay windows were reflected on the opposite wall near the bed and looked like train windows! We also live near a freeway and the car sounds could be misheard as a moving train.

The main task is not to argue or become upset because the person is talking crazy. The goal is to help them feel safe and accepted. We should ask, "When language skills become problematic, then how are people with dementia going to communicate their unmet needs?" "How can they let us know what they are feeling or experiencing in a particular situation?"

We all know communication is more than speaking certain words. It's the way we say it that determines how we take the message. This, of course, is the nonverbal communication we all use. If we say, "I believe you" but roll our eyes to someone else in the room, then the person is not going to believe us.

Dr. Mark Coggins (Coggins 2015) suggests we use the terms "behavioral expressions" instead of "behavioral problems." We are more likely to deal with the situation differently. We will consider the behavior as an expression of the situation. We can change the cause, whether it is environmental, personal, or physical, and decrease the unwanted behavior.

He gives a succinct list of communication tips in his article:
- Use a calm voice
- Offer no more than two choice
- Avoid open-ended questions, and keep communication simple.
- Consider the person's nonverbal expressions as unmet needs and attend to those needs promptly.
- Create structured daily routines that are consistent and predictable.
- Keep the individual engaged with activities that match interests and capabilities.
- Use cueing strategies such as touch and verbal directions.

Most sources explain the diagnostic workup and evaluation the person according to her own history. This will take into account internal and external factors that can increase severity of the dementia.

There are things we should consider when there is a sudden change in behavior. The following outline highlights possible reasons for behavior changes. The main reason delirium should be addressed first is because it can be reversed with appropriate treatment quickly.

## A. Delirium

1. Infections — check for worsening cough, fever, urinary symptoms, sore throat or earache.

2. Medications — look to see if new medications have been added to her medical regimen, avoid using antihistamines which can cause confusion.

3. Metabolic — this would be a worsening of their diabetes, becoming dehydrated, or because of diarrhea or vomiting have an imbalance of their electrolytes, like sodium and potassium.

## B. Environmental

1. Look around for confusing shadows that may occur late in the afternoon

2. Poor lighting, especially in the afternoon, can cause a confusion and agitation known as sun downing

3. Becoming overly stimulated with television or radio sounds, too many people talking at once, being out of their normal environment and getting fatigued

4. TV and radio program can create illusions, that is, the person believes the program is speaking to them personally.

## C. Personal history

1. It's important to know their past because certain triggers (people or situations) should be avoided if it causes mental agitation.

2. We need to know what their level of understanding is at this point. They may find some situations too difficult to process.

3. We should know what things, words, gestures will calm them. It could be their favorite music, or a prayer, or a back rub.

### D. Interpersonal relationship

1. As verbal ability decreases, they become more sensitive to the feelings of others. They can quickly pick up on someone else's anxiety or anger.

2. They are very good at realizing when the words are not in sync with the person's emotions. If a person is sad about something but tells the person with dementia that he is okay, then this becomes a confusing situation for the one with dementia.

### E. Psychological manifestations

1. Depression should be treated because they will act out on the sad feelings. They may stop participating or want to stay in bed. Then this situation becomes a constant source for an argument.

2. Anxiety will manifest as agitation or fear. Medications that treat anxiety can sometimes causes the opposite effect. I found that a very small dose of Ativan would help break a panic attack in Tom so he would start talking to me again.

3. Hallucinations occur when they see people or things that you cannot see. Sometimes the hallucination will come out of a dream or a triggered memory. If it is harmless, just go with it. It's not essential to try to get them to see it isn't real. If the hallucination could cause an increase in agitation or anger, then sometimes re-directing or distracting will help the person move past it. It helps to remove what may be stimulating the hallucination if possible.

4. Misidentifying (Illusion) — the person may see a scrap of paper on the floor and say, "People shouldn't be careless with their money." The simplest solution is to pick up the paper and say, "I agree. I'll make sure the money is returned."

# Simple Do's and Don'ts

**Don'ts**

1. Reason with words or arguments — This will usually cause more confusion and agitation.

2. Insist on reality — they can become more confused and sometimes have to relive a sad experience. A man wanted to see his wife, who had died 5 years before. The assistant at first said, "Your wife died 5 years ago, don't you remember?" The man began to cry over the death of his wife. Another day, the man again asked to see his wife. This time the assistant said, "I know she loves you very much. But it's getting chilly. Let's go and get you a sweater before we find her." On the way to getting his sweater they went by the activity room where someone was singing songs. The assistant took him in and he started singing the songs. Instead of having him relive the loss of his wife daily, isn't it better to redirect him?

**Dos**

1. Support the emotion behind the hallucinations

2. With fear — reassure in concrete terms and gestures

3. With joy or happiness — participate in what they feel

4. With love — reciprocate with hugs and words of friendship

5. With aggression or anger —

    A. Reassure

    B. Apologize for "apparent" problem

C. Distract by moving in another direction emotionally or physically

D. Leave the room and person, if the anger is directed at you, for 5-10 minutes. When you return, return with a smile and something positive to say

E. If behavior continues to occur under certain conditions that cannot be altered, then consider getting medical treatment for anxiety or depression

It is so important to realize the uniqueness of *this* individual's history and personality.

This allows personal and individual care as "one size does *not* fit all."

I discovered a handout by Liz Ayres called *Compassionate Communication*. I would like to share the entire handbook with you because I like the way she organizes the concepts.

A wonderful, helpful handout to help you speak with a memory impaired person.

DON'T

Don't reason.
Don't argue.
Don't confront.
Don't remind them they forget.
Don't question recent memory.
Don't take it personally.

DO

Give short, one sentence explanations.
Allow plenty of time for comprehension, then triple it.
Repeat instructions or sentences exactly the same way.
Eliminate 'but' from your vocabulary; substitute 'nevertheless.'
Avoid insistence. Try again later.
Agree with them or distract them to a different subject or activity.
Accept blame when something's wrong (even if it's fantasy).
Leave the room, if necessary, to avoid confrontations.
Respond to feelings rather than words.
Be patient and cheerful and reassuring. Do go with the flow.
Practice 100% forgiveness. Memory loss progresses daily.
My appeal to you:
**Please** *elevate your level of generosity and graciousness*

<u>Remember to be kind by being aware of the following concepts:</u>

**You can't control memory loss**, only your reaction to it.
Compassionate communication will significantly heighten quality of life.

**They are not crazy or lazy**.
They say normal things, and do normal things, for a memory impaired, dementia individual. If they were deliberately trying to exasperate you, they would have a different diagnosis. Forgive them...always. For example: they don't hide things; they protect them in safe places...And then forget. *Don't take 'stealing' accusations personally.*

**Their disability is memory loss**.
Asking them to remember is like asking a blind person to read. Don't' ask and don't test memory! A loss of this magnitude reduces the capacity to reason.
Example: "Did you take your pills?" "What did you do today?"
Expecting them to be reasonable or to accept your conclusion is unrealistic. Don't try to reason or convince them.
Example: "You need a shower." "Day care will be fun." "You can't live alone."
Give a one sentence explanation or search for creative solutions. Memory loss produces unpredictable emotions, thought, and behavior, which you can alleviate by resolving all issues **peacefully**. *Don't argue, correct, contradict, confront, blames, or insist.*

**They are scared all the time**.

Each patient reacts differently to fear. They may become passive, uncooperative, hostile, angry, agitated, verbally abusive, or physically combative. They may even do them all at different times, or alternate between them. Anxiety may compel them to shadow you (follow everywhere). Anxiety compels them to resist changes in routine, even pleasant ones.

*Your goal is to reduce anxiety whenever possible. Also, they can't remember your reassurances. Keep saying them."*

In *Diagnosis, Management and Treatment of Dementia* published by the American Medical Association (2012) there is a succinct table of ways to say things to help the person with dementia understand.

| Speech style | |
| --- | --- |
| Get patient's attention before speaking | Limit the use of pronouns e.g. he, she |
| Lightly touch hand to (re) gain attention | Limit colloquialisms as the patient may interpret them literally. |
| Use direct statements, limiting technical jargon or lengthy explanations | Place modifiers after nouns and provide a choice e.g. "Do you have pain...sharp or dull?" |
| Try yes/no questions for memory prompting | Speak calmly, slowly and clearly, pausing to stress words and highlight information |
| Place important information at the start of the sentence | Speak slightly louder and at a lower pitch if patient is hearing impaired |

In the following pages Ms. Ayres gives scenarios so you can imagine certain situations and how to handle them.

**Don't reason**

| Patient: | | What doctor's appointment? There's nothing wrong with me. |
|---|---|---|
| **Don't** | *Reason* | You've been seeing the doctor every three months for the last two years. It's written on the calendar and I told you about it yesterday and this morning. |
| **Do** | *Short explanation* | It's just a regular check-up. |
| | *Accept blames* | I'm sorry if I forgot to tell you. |

**Don't question recent memory**

| Patient: | | Hello, Mary. I see you've brought a friend with you. |
|---|---|---|
| **Don't'** | *Question memory* | Hi. Mom. You remember Eric, don't you? What did you do today? |
| **Do** | *Short explanation* | Hi, Mom. You look wonderful! This is Eric. We work together. |

## Don't take it personally!

| Patient | | Who are you? Where's my husband? |
|---|---|---|
| **Don't** | *Take it personally* | What do you mean — who's your husband? I am! |
| **Do** | *Go with the flow, reassure* | He'll be here for dinner. |
| | *Distract* | How about some milk and cookies? Would you like chocolate chip or oatmeal? |

## Do repeat exactly

| Patient | | I'm going to the store for a newspaper. |
|---|---|---|
| **Don't** | *Repeat differently* | Please put your shoes on. You'll need to put your shoes on. |
| **Do** | *Repeat exactly* | Please put your shoes on. Please put your shoes on. |

**Do eliminate "but",          substitute "nevertheless"**

| Patient | | I don't want to eat chicken. |
|---------|------------------|------------------------------|
| **Don't** | *Say "but"* | I know chicken's not your favorite food, but its' what we're having for dinner. |
| **Do** | *Say "nevertheless"* | I know chicken's not your favorite food, (smile) *nevertheless* I'd appreciate it if you'd eat a little bit. |

**Don't argue**

| Patient | | I didn't write this check for $500. Someone at the bank is forging my signature. |
|---------|------------------|------------------------------|
| **Don'ts** | *Argue* | What' Don't be silly! The bank wouldn't be forging your signature. |
| **Do** | *Respond to feelings* | That's a scary thought. |
| | *Reassure* | I'll make sure they don't do that. |
| | *Distract* | Would you help me fold the towels? |

## Don't Confront

| Patient | | "*Nobody's going to make decisions for me. You can go now...and don't come back.* |
|---|---|---|
| **Don't** | *Confront* | I'm not going anywhere and you can't remember enough to make your own decisions. |
| **Do** | *Accept blame or respond to feelings* | I'm sorry this is a tough time. |
| | *Reassure* | I love you and we're going to get through this together. |
| | *Distract* | You know what? Don has a new job. He's really excited about it. |

## Don't' remind them they forgot

| Patient | | "*Joe hasn't called for a long time. I hope he's okay.*" |
|---|---|---|
| **Don't** | *Remind* | Joe called yesterday and you talked to him for 15 minutes. |
| **Do** | *Reassure* | You really like talking to Joe, don't you? |
| | *Distract* | Let's call him when we get back from our walk. |

So as we have seen in this chapter, there are various conditions and situations that can trigger a behavioral expression. It can be the person with dementia's mental state, such as depression or anxiety. The other factors that come into play are environmental and interpersonal.

It is important there is emotional synchronicity, especially when a person's language ability is compromised. So, if what I'm saying isn't what I'm feeling it will cause confusion and rejection in the person with dementia.

We are all aware of nonverbal cues but it is truly recognized by someone with dementia. If I am feeling tense, anxious or uncertain, then the person with dementia will hone in on these feelings and won't listen to what I am trying to tell him. If I feel positive so I come across friendly, open and calm, then this will be accepted and the person with dementia will also respond in a positive way.

# Chapter Four

Ways to Help
The Individual with Dementia
By Volunteering
As a Dementia Friend
Resources
References

I hope after reading this chapter your comfort level will increase when assisting people with dementia. There are times we all find we don't know what to say or how to help.

If you notice someone appears to be wandering and looking confused there are several things you can do:

1. Ask in a friendly way if you can help.

2. Ask them if you can check to see if they are wearing a special wrist band or pendant. This is to see if they have been registered with Medic Alert-Safe Return. By calling the number on the band their caregiver can be identified.

3. Ask if they are with a friend or family member, and help them locate that person by taking them to a security guard or employee of the store to over-head page the person they are with.

4. It is important to respond to their emotions and not their words. They may be frightened and because of this have more trouble finding the right words.

5. While waiting for their companion talk about neutral subjects, i.e. nature, people walking by, etc

6. Many of us automatically ask about occupations or professions. But this can cause anxiety since they may think they should know that but can't remember. Let them take the lead about professions and jobs.

And remember: It takes about 60 seconds for someone with dementia to process a question so give them time to respond.

If you are interested in helping those with dementia so they do not feel forgotten, then you can volunteer to become a friend to someone in a Day Care or nursing home.

If there is a Memory Café in your area, see about volunteering to serve the coffee or plan activities for those that attend.

I have compiled a list of resources I found helpful. I'm sure there are many more books to be read and websites to be seen. If there is a particular website or book you have found helpful, I would like to hear about it on my blog.

There are a couple of books that I found personally helpful in understanding the world of the person with Alzheimer's dementia. I have recommended them to friends. They feel more comfortable talking and helping their friends with dementia after reading the book.

The first book that I found not only helpful but also hopeful was *Learning to Speak Alzheimer's* by Joanne Koenig Coste.

I also downloaded an e-book called *Understanding the Dementia Experience* by Jennifer Ghent-Fuller.

Finally, a book that was ahead of its time: *Dementia Reconsidered* by Tom Kitwood. He addressed the importance of treating people with dementia with respect and acknowledging their personhood and individuality. The following pages will include other recommendations in a table form.

| Website address | Note |
| --- | --- |
| Educational sites & research | |
| www.helpguide.org | Give links to understand diagnosis of different syndromes |
| www.alzheimersreadingroo m.com | Alzheimer's Reading Room |
| www.dementiacare.com | Give strategies for caregivers & families |
| www.fightdementia.org/au | Fight Alzheimer's |
| www.medicinenet.com/deme nta/article.html | Medicine Net – articles about dementia |
| www.ninds.nih.gov/disorder/ dementias/de | National Institute of Neurological Disorders |
| www.alzbabes.org | B. A.B.E.S – supports Research at UC San Diego |
| www.ucdmc.ucdavis.edu/alz heimers | Alzheimer's Disease Center – UC Davis Health System |
| www.memory.ucsf.edu | UCSF Memory & Aging Center |
| www.svalz.stanford.edu | Stanford/VA Alzheimer's Research Center – Stanford University |

| Website address | Notes |
| --- | --- |
| Cognition programs | |
| www.aarp.org/health/brain-health/brain_games | Entertainment link – brain games |
| www.health.gove.au/dementia | Department of Health & Aging (Australia) |
| www.proprofs.com/games | |
| www.fitbrains.com/brain-games | Fit Brains by Rosetta Stone ($) |
| www.gamesforthbrain.com | Games for the Brain |
| Games.yahoo.com | |
| www.lumosity | Lumosity (4) |
| www.brainhq.com | Brain HQ (by Posit Science $) |

| Website address | Notes |
| --- | --- |
| Legal & home care services | |
| www.caregiver.org | Family Caregiver Alliance (good contact for elder-care lawyer to draw up a will, durable power, etc) |
| www.ourparentsplace.com | Out Parents Place – home services |
| www.placeformom.com | Gives local addresses of assisted living, home care |
| www.lotsahelpinghands.com | Allows caregivers to co-ordinate care; runs slowly but can plan a workable schedule |
| www.alz.org | Alzheimer's Association – 800-272-3900 (24 hr hotline) |
| www.medicalert.org/safereturn | Safe Return program |

| | through Medic Alert |
|---|---|

| **Books** | | |
|---|---|---|
| Bazan-Salazar, Emilia C. | Alzheimer's Activities That Stimulate the Mind | 2005 |
| Ghent-Fuller, Jennifer | Understanding the Dementia Experience | 2012 |
| Gruetzner, Howard | Alzheimer's: A Caregiver's Guide and Source Book | 1992 |
| Kitwood, Tom | Dementia Reconsidered:  The Person Comes First | 1997 |
| Koenig-Coste, Joanne | Learning to Speak Alzheimer's | 2003 |
| Mace, Nancy L. Rabins, Peter V | The 36-Hour Day, 4th Edition | 2006 |

# References

# References

*7 Stages of Alzheimer's.* (e.d.). Retrieved from Alzheimer's
    Associate: www.alz.org

American Medical Association. (1999). *Diagnosis, Management
    and Treatment of Dementia.* Chicago: AMA.

Association, A. (2014). Top Ten Warning Signs of Alzheimer's
    Dementia. Retrieved from www.alz.org

Ayres, L. (2013). Compassionate Communication with the
    Memory Impaired.

Bashore, P. G. (2006). *Module 5: Neuroanatomy of Alzheimer's
    Disease.* Retrieved from www.home.comcast.net/-
    bashorechanges.html

Black, K. P. (2014). Alzheimer's Disease And Related
    Neurocognitive Disorders. Brockton, MA: Western
    Schools. Retrieved from www.westernschools.com

Coggins, Mark D. (2015). Behavioral Expressions in Dementia
    Patients. *Today's Geriatric Medicine,* Jan/Feb 2015, 6-9.

Coste, J. K. (2003). *Learning to Speak Alzheimer's.* Boston:
    Houghton Mifflin Company.

*Executive function.* (n.d.). Retrieved from Encyclopedia of
    Mental Disorders:
    http://www.minddisorders.com/Del-Fi/Executive-
    function.html

Heyman, A., Wilkinson, W., & Hurwitz, B. e. (1987). Early-
    onset Alzheimer's disease: clinical predictors of
    institutionalization and death. *Neurology, 37*(6), 980-984.

Howard, M. E. (2014). Understanding Dementia. *Understanding Dementia* (p. 15). Oakland: Institute for Natural Resources.

Hughes, C., Berg, L., Danziger, W., & al, e. (1982). A new clinical scale for the staging of dementia. *British Journal of Psychiatry, 140*, 566-572.

Kitwood, T. (1997). *Dementia Reconsidered.* Buckingham, England: Open University Press.

Morris, J. (1993). The Clinical Dementia Rating (CDR) current version and scoring rules. *Neurology, 43*(11), 2412-2414.

# Conclusion

This final chapter will be to encourage you to support the Dementia Friend Movement. You can reach out and help those with dementia as well as being a support to the caregiver. I am offering the Dementia Friend kits free so people will sign up to help. As I mention on my website, I hope everyone will take time to attend a talk about dementia. Alzheimer's Association offers lectures in different cities. They also have links on their website with more information about this disease.

I will be speaking at various locations in the San Francisco Bay Area. The times and locations of my talks will be given on the website in the Dementia Friend link.

Donations on my website www.memorydaybyday.org will help support the nonprofit company, Memory DayByDay, in offering the Dementia Friend kit as well as the programs to help those with early-onset Alzheimer's dementia.

Memory DayByDay is currently seeking nonprofit 501 ( c ) 3 certification so that all donations can be tax deductible. I will post the date of this certification on my website once it occurs.

Other ways of helping to spread the news is to tell friends and family members about signing up to receive a Dementia Friend kit. This is also something that may help someone newly diagnosed with Alzheimer's dementia and their caregiver.

On the website is a list of Resources I have found helpful. I'm sure there are many more to be read and seen. If there is a particular website or book you have found helpful I would like to hear about it on my blog.

I look forward to hearing from anyone who wants to help advance awareness to increase respect and care for people with dementia.

I leave you with one more story of Tom which highlights the reasons to help support people with dementia.

One day I came into our living room and saw Tom sitting in his chair looking sad. I asked, "Tom, how are you doing?" He looked at me and said quietly, " I don't think anyone remembers me."

His feelings completely changed after we returned from his high school class reunion. He saw and recognized many of his friends from his teenage years and never again felt he had been forgotten.

You too can make this kind of difference to someone with dementia.

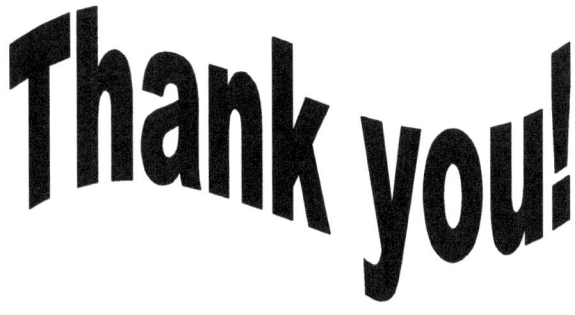

Thank you!